# Quick and Easy Mediterranean Recipes

## Super Delicious Recipes for your everday Healthy meals

Lara Dillard

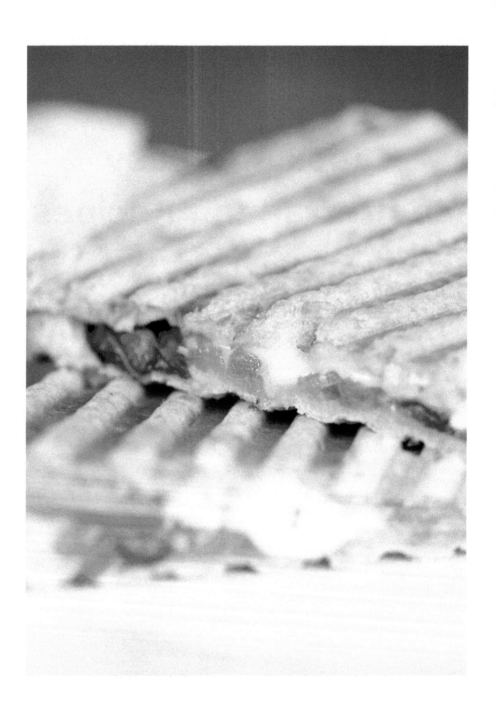

# Table of Contents

# Caprese Grilled Cheese

**Difficulty Level: 2/5**

**Preparation time: 10 minutes**

**Cooking time: 10 minutes**

**Servings: 4**

## Ingredients:

4 Versatile Sandwich Rounds

8 tablespoons jarred pesto

4 ounces fresh mozzarella cheese, cut into 4 round slices

1 Roma tomato or small slicing tomato, cut into 4 slices

4 tablespoons extra-virgin olive oil

## Directions:

In a microwave-safe ramekin, combine the almond flour, olive oil, egg, rosemary (if using), baking powder, and salt. Mix well with a fork.

Microwave for 90 seconds on high.

Slide a knife around the edges of ramekin and flip to remove the bread.

Slice in half with a serrated knife if you want to use it to make a sandwich.

**Nutrition:**

Per serving

Calories: 232

Total fat: 22g

Sodium: 450mg

Total Carbohydrates: 1g

Fiber: 0g

Protein: 8g

# Riced Cauliflower

**Difficulty Level: 2/5**

**Preparation time: 5 minutes**

**Cooking time: 10 minutes**

**Servings: 6-8**

## Ingredients:

1 small head cauliflower, broken into florets

¼ cup extra-virgin olive oil

2 garlic cloves, finely minced

1½ teaspoons salt

½ teaspoon freshly ground black pepper

## Directions:

Place the florets in a food processor and pulse several times, until the cauliflower is the consistency of rice or couscous.

In a large skillet, heat the olive oil over medium-high heat. Add the cauliflower, garlic, salt, and pepper and sauté for 5 minutes, just to take the crunch out but not enough to let the cauliflower become soggy.

Remove the cauliflower from the skillet and place in a bowl until ready to use. Toss with chopped herbs and additional olive oil for a simple side, top with sautéed veggies and protein, or use in your favorite recipe.

**Nutrition:**

Per serving

Calories: 92

Total fat: 9g

Sodium: 595mg

Total Carbohydrates: 3g

Fiber: 1g

Protein: 1g

# Greek Chicken and "Rice" Soup with Artichokes

**Difficulty Level: 2/5**

**Preparation time: 10 minutes**

**Cooking time: 15 minutes**

**Servings: 4**

**Ingredients:**

4 cups chicken stock

2 cups Riced Cauliflower, divided

2 large egg yolks

¼ cup freshly squeezed lemon juice (about 2 lemons)

¾ cup extra-virgin olive oil, divided

8 ounces cooked chicken, coarsely chopped

1 (13.75-ounce) can artichoke hearts, drained and quartered

¼ cup chopped fresh dill

## Directions:

In a large saucepan, bring the stock to a low boil. Reduce the heat to low and simmer, covered.

Transfer 1 cup of the hot stock to a blender or food processor. Add ½ cup raw riced cauliflower, the egg yolks, and lemon juice and purée. While the processor or blender is running, stream in ½ cup olive oil and blend until smooth.

Whisking constantly, pour the purée into the simmering stock until well blended together and smooth. Add the chicken and artichokes and simmer until thickened slightly, 8 to 10 minutes. Stir in the dill and remaining 1½ cups riced cauliflower. Serve warm, drizzled with the remaining ¼ cup olive oil.

## Nutrition:

Per serving

Calories: 566

Total fat: 46g

Sodium: 754mg

Total Carbohydrates: 14g

Fiber: 7g

Protein: 24g

# Citrus Asparagus with Pistachios

**Difficulty Level: 2/5**

**Preparation time: 10 minutes**

**Cooking time: 15 minutes**

**Servings: 4**

**Ingredients:**

5 tablespoons extra-virgin olive oil, divided

Zest and juice of 2 clementines or 1 orange (about ¼ cup juice and 1 tablespoon zest)

Zest and juice of 1 lemon

1 tablespoon red wine vinegar

1 teaspoon salt, divided

¼ teaspoon freshly ground black pepper

½ cup shelled pistachios

1 pound fresh asparagus

1 tablespoon water

## Directions:

In a small bowl, whisk together 4 tablespoons olive oil, the clementine and lemon juices and zests, vinegar, ½ teaspoon salt, and pepper. Set aside.

In a medium dry skillet, toast the pistachios over medium-high heat until lightly browned, 2 to 3 minutes, being careful not to let them burn. Transfer to a cutting board and coarsely chop. Set aside.

Trim the rough ends off the asparagus, usually the last 1 to 2 inches of each spear. In a skillet, heat the remaining 1 tablespoon olive oil over medium-high heat. Add the asparagus and sauté for 2 to 3 minutes. Sprinkle with the remaining ½ teaspoon salt and add the water. Reduce the heat to medium-low, cover, and cook until tender, another 2 to 4 minutes, depending on the thickness of the spears.

Transfer the cooked asparagus to a serving dish. Add the pistachios to the dressing and whisk to combine. Pour the dressing over the warm asparagus and toss to coat.

**Nutrition:**

Per serving

Calories: 284

Total fat: 24g

Sodium: 594mg

Total Carbohydrates: 11g

Fiber: 4g

Protein: 6g

# Garlicky Shrimp with Mushrooms

**Difficulty Level: 2/5**

**Preparation time: 10 minutes**

**Cooking time: 15 minutes**

**Servings: 4**

**Ingredients:**

1 pound peeled and deveined fresh shrimp

1 teaspoon salt

1 cup extra-virgin olive oil

8 large garlic cloves, thinly sliced

4 ounces sliced mushrooms (shiitake, baby bella, or button)

½ teaspoon red pepper flakes

¼ cup chopped fresh flat-leaf Italian parsley

Zucchini Noodles or Riced Cauliflower, for serving

## Directions:

In a small bowl, whisk together 4 tablespoons olive oil, the clementine and lemon juices and zests, vinegar, ½ teaspoon salt, and pepper. Set aside.

In a medium dry skillet, toast the pistachios over medium-high heat until lightly browned, 2 to 3 minutes, being careful not to let them burn. Transfer to a cutting board and coarsely chop. Set aside.

Trim the rough ends off the asparagus, usually the last 1 to 2 inches of each spear. In a skillet, heat the remaining 1 tablespoon olive oil over medium-high heat. Add the asparagus and sauté for 2 to 3 minutes. Sprinkle with the remaining ½ teaspoon salt and add the water. Reduce the heat to medium-low, cover, and cook until tender, another 2 to 4 minutes, depending on the thickness of the spears.

Transfer the cooked asparagus to a serving dish. Add the pistachios to the dressing and whisk to combine. Pour the dressing over the warm asparagus and toss to coat.

**Nutrition:**

Per serving

Calories: 284

Total fat: 24g

Sodium: 594mg

Total Carbohydrates: 11g

Fiber: 4g

Protein: 6g

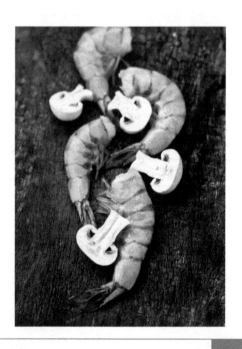

# Zucchini Noodles

**Difficulty Level: 1/5**

**Preparation time: 5 minutes**

**Cooking time: 0 minutes**

**Servings: 4**

**Ingredients:**

2 medium to large zucchini

**Directions:**

Cut off and discard the ends of each zucchini and, using a spiralizer set to the smallest setting, spiralize the zucchini to create zoodles.

To serve, simply place a ½ cup or so of spiralized zucchini into the bottom of each bowl and spoon a hot sauce over top to "cook" the zoodles to al dente consistency. Use with any of your favorite sauces, or just toss with warmed pesto for a simple and quick meal.

**Nutrition:**

Per serving

Calories: 48

Total fat: 1g

Sodium: 7mg

Total Carbohydrates: 7g

Fiber: 3g

Protein: 6g

# Cod with Parsley Pistou

**Difficulty Level: 2/5**

**Preparation time: 15 minutes**

**Cooking time: 10 minutes**

**Servings: 4**

**Ingredients:**

1 cup packed roughly chopped fresh flat-leaf Italian parsley

1 to 2 small garlic cloves, minced

Zest and juice of 1 lemon

1 teaspoon salt

½ teaspoon freshly ground black pepper

1 cup extra-virgin olive oil, divided

1 pound cod fillets, cut into 4 equal-sized pieces

**Directions:**

In a food processer, combine the parsley, garlic, lemon zest and juice, salt, and pepper. Pulse to chop well.

While the food processor is running, slowly stream in ¾ cup olive oil until well combined. Set aside.

In a large skillet, heat the remaining ¼ cup olive oil over medium-high heat. Add the cod fillets, cover, and cook 4 to 5 minutes on each side, or until cooked through. Thicker fillets may require a bit more cooking time. Remove from the heat and keep warm.

Add the pistou to the skillet and heat over medium-low heat. Return the cooked fish to the skillet, flipping to coat in the sauce. Serve warm, covered with pistou.

**Nutrition:**

Calories: 581

Total Fat: 55g,

Total Carbohydrates: 3g,

Net Carbohydrates: 2g,

Fiber: 1g,

Protein: 21g;

Sodium: 652mg

# Rosemary-Lemon Snapper Baked

# in Parchment

**Difficulty Level: 2/5**

**Preparation time: 15 minutes**

**Cooking time: 15 minutes**

**Servings: 4**

**Ingredients:**

1¼ pounds fresh red snapper fillet, cut into two equal pieces

2 lemons, thinly sliced

6 to 8 sprigs fresh rosemary, stems removed or 1 to 2 tablespoons dried rosemary

½ cup extra-virgin olive oil

6 garlic cloves, thinly sliced

1 teaspoon salt

½ teaspoon freshly ground black pepper

**Directions:**

Preheat the oven to 425°F.

Place two large sheets of parchment (about twice the size of each piece of fish) on the counter. Place 1 piece of fish in the center of each sheet.

Top the fish pieces with lemon slices and rosemary leaves.

In a small bowl, combine the olive oil, garlic, salt, and pepper. Drizzle the oil over each piece of fish.

5 . Top each piece of fish with a second large sheet of parchment and starting on a long side, fold the paper up to about 1 inch from the fish. Repeat on the remaining sides, going in a clockwise direction. Fold in each corner once to secure.

Place both parchment pouches on a baking sheet and bake until the fish is cooked through, 10 to 12 minutes.

**Nutrition:**

Calories: 390,

Total Fat: 29g,

Total Carbohydrates: 3g,

Net Carbohydrates: 3g,

Fiber: 0g,

Protein: 29g;

Sodium: 674mg

# Shrimp in Creamy Pesto over Zoodles

**Difficulty Level: 2/5**

**Preparation time: 10 minutes**

**Cooking time: 10 minutes**

**Servings: 4**

**Ingredients:**

1 pound peeled and deveined fresh shrimp

Salt

Freshly ground black pepper

2 tablespoons extra-virgin olive oil

½ small onion, slivered

8 ounces store-bought jarred pesto

¾ cup crumbled goat or feta cheese, plus more for serving

6 cups Zucchini Noodles (from about 2 large zucchini), for serving

¼ cup chopped flat-leaf Italian parsley, for garnish

**Directions:**

In a bowl, season the shrimp with salt and pepper and set aside.

In a large skillet, heat the olive oil over medium-high heat. Sauté the onion until just golden, 5 to 6 minutes.

Reduce the heat to low and add the pesto and cheese, whisking to combine and melt the cheese. Bring to a low simmer and add the shrimp. Reduce the heat back to low and cover. Cook until the shrimp is cooked through and pink, another 3 to 4 minutes.

Serve warm over Zucchini Noodles, garnishing with chopped parsley and additional crumbled cheese, if desired.

**Nutrition:**

Calories: 491,

Total Fat: 35g,

Total Carbohydrates: 15g,

Net Carbohydrates: 11g,

Fiber: 4g,

Protein: 29g;

Sodium: 870mg

# Nut-Crusted Baked Fish

**Difficulty Level: 2/5**

**Preparation time: 10 minutes**

**Cooking time: 20 minutes**

**Servings: 4**

**Ingredients:**

½ cup extra-virgin olive oil, divided

1 pound flaky white fish (such as cod, haddock, or halibut), skin removed

½ cup shelled finely chopped pistachios

½ cup ground flaxseed

Zest and juice of 1 lemon, divided

1 teaspoon ground cumin

1 teaspoon ground allspice

½ teaspoon salt (use 1 teaspoon if pistachios are unsalted)

¼ teaspoon freshly ground black pepper

**Directions:**

Preheat the oven to 400°F.

Line a baking sheet with parchment paper or aluminum foil and drizzle 2 tablespoons olive oil over the sheet, spreading to coat the bottom evenly.

Cut the fish into 4 equal pieces and place on the prepared baking sheet.

In a small bowl, combine the pistachios, flaxseed, lemon zest, cumin, allspice, salt, and pepper. Drizzle in ¼ cup olive oil and stir well.

Divide the nut mixture evenly atop the fish pieces. Drizzle the lemon juice and remaining 2 tablespoons oil over the fish and bake until cooked through, 15 to 20 minutes, depending on the thickness of the fish.

**Nutrition:**

Calories: 509,

Total Fat: 41g,

Total Carbohydrates: 9g,

Net Carbohydrates: 3g,

Fiber: 6g,

Protein: 26g;

Sodium: 331mg

# Pesto Walnut Noodles

**Difficulty Level: 2/5**

**Preparation time: 10 minutes**

**Cooking time: 15 minutes**

**Servings: 4**

**Ingredients:**

4 Zucchini, Made into Zoodles

¼ Cup Olive Oil, Divided

½ Teaspoon Crushed Red Pepper

2 Cloves Garlic, Minced & Divided

¼ Teaspoon Black Pepper

¼ Teaspoon sea Salt

2 Tablespoons Parmesan Cheese, Grated & Divided

1 Cup Basil, Fresh & Packed

¾ Cup Walnut Pieces, Divided

## Directions:

Start by making your zucchini noodles by using a spiralizer to get ribbons. Combine your zoodles with a minced garlic clove and tablespoon of oil. Season with salt and pepper and crushed red pepper. Set it to the side.

Get out a large skillet and heat a ½ a tablespoon of oil over medium-high heat. Add in half of your zoodles, cooking for five minutes. You will need to stir every minute or so. Repeat with another ½ a tablespoon of oil and your remaining zoodles.

Make your pesto while your zoodles cook. Put your garlic clove, a tablespoon or parmesan, basil leaves and ¼ cup of walnuts in your food processor. Season with salt and pepper if desired, and drizzle the remaining two tablespoons of oil in until completely blended.

Add the pesto to your zoodles, topping with remaining walnuts and parmesan to serve.

## Nutrition:

Calories: 301

Protein: 7 Grams

Fat: 28 Grams

Carbohydrates: 11 Grams

Sodium: 160 mg

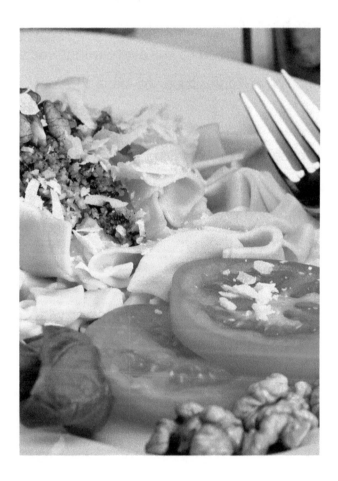

# Tomato Tabbouleh

**Difficulty Level: 2/5**

**Preparation time: 10 minutes**

**Cooking time: 20 minutes**

**Servings: 4**

**Ingredients:**

8 Beefsteak Tomatoes

½ Cup Water

3 Tablespoons Olive Oil, Divided

½ Cup Whole Wheat Couscous, Uncooked

1 ½ Cups Parsley, Fresh & Minced

2 Scallions Chopped

1/3 Cup Mint, Fresh & Minced

Sea Salt & Black Pepper to Taste

1 Lemon

4 Teaspoons Honey, Raw

1/3 Cup Almonds, Chopped

**Directions:**

Start by heating your oven to 400 degrees. Take your tomato and slice the top off each one before scooping the flesh out. Put the tops flesh and seeds in a mixing bowl.

Get out a baking dish before adding in a tablespoon of oil to grease it. Place your tomatoes in the dish, and then cover your dish with foil.

Now you will make your couscous while your tomatoes cook. Bring the water to a boil using a saucepan and then add the couscous in and cover. Remove it from heat, and allow it to sit for five minutes. Fluff it with a fork.

Chop your tomato flesh and tops up, and then drain the excess water using a colander. Measure a cup of your chopped tomatoes and place them back in the mixing bowl. Mix with mint scallions, pepper, salt and parsley.

Zest your lemon into the bowl, and then half the lemon. Squeeze the lemon juice in, and mix well.

Add your tomato mix to the couscous.

Carefully remove your tomatoes from the oven and then divide your tabbouleh among your tomatoes. Cover the pan with foil and then put it in the oven. Cook for another eight to ten minutes. Your tomatoes should be firm but still tender.

Drizzle with honey and top with almonds before serving.

**Nutrition:**

Calories: 314

Protein: 8 Grams

Fat: 15 Grams

Carbohydrates: 41 Grams

Sodium: 141

# Lemon Faro Bowl

**Difficulty Level: 2/5**

**Preparation time: 10 minutes**

**Cooking time: 15 minutes**

**Servings: 6**

**Ingredients:**

1 Tablespoon + 2 Teaspoons Olive Oil, Divided

1 Cup Onion, Chopped

2 Cloves Garlic, Minced

1 Carrot, Shredded

2 Cups Vegetable Broth, Low Sodium

1 Cup Pearled Faro

2 Avocados, Peeled, Pitted & Sliced

1 Lemon, Small

Sea Salt to Taste

## Directions:

Start by placing a saucepan over medium-high heat. Add in a tablespoon of oil and then throw in your onion once the oil is hot. Cook for about five minutes, stirring frequently to keep it from burning.

Add in your carrot and garlic. Allow it to cook for about another minute while you continue to stir.

Add in your broth and faro. Allow it to come to a boil and adjust your heat to high to help. Once it boils, lower it to medium-low and cover your saucepan. Let it simmer for twenty minutes. The faro should be al dente and plump.

Pour the faro into a bowl and add in your avocado and zest. Drizzle with your remaining oil and add in your lemon wedges.

## Nutrition:

Calories: 279

Protein: 7 Grams

Fat: 14 Grams

Carbohydrates: 36 Grams

Sodium: 118 mg

# Chickpea & Red Pepper Delight

**Difficulty Level: 2/5**

**Preparation time: 15 minutes**

**Cooking time: 15 minutes**

**Servings: 3**

**Ingredients:**

1 Red Bell Pepper, Diced

2 Cups Water

4 Sun-Dried Tomatoes

¼ Cup Red Wine Vinegar

2 Tablespoon Olive Oil

2 Cloves Garlic, Chopped

29 Ounces Chickpeas, Canned, Drained & Rinsed

½ Cup Parsley, Chopped **/** Sea Salt to Taste

**Directions:**

Get a baking sheet and put your red bell pepper on it with the skin side up.

Bake for eight minutes. Your skin should bubble, and then place it in a bag to seal it.

Remove your bell peppers in about ten minutes, and then slice it into thin slices.

Get out two cups of water and pour it in a bowl. Microwave for four minutes and add in your sundried tomatoes, letting them sit for ten minutes. Drain them before slicing into thin strips. Mix your red wine vinegar and garlic with your olive oil. Ross your roasted red bell pepper with parsley, sun dried tomatoes, and chickpeas. Season with salt before serving.

**Nutrition:**

Calories: 195

Protein: 9.3 Grams

Fat: 8.5 Grams

Carbohydrates: 25.5 Grams

Sodium: 142 mg

# Chickpea Salad

**Difficulty Level: 2/5**

**Preparation time: 10 minutes**

**Cooking time: 0 minutes**

**Servings: 6**

**Ingredients:**

28 ounces chickpeas, drained

½ red onion, chopped fine

2 cucumbers, chopped fine

¼ cup olive oil

2 lemons, juiced

1 lemon, zested

1 tablespoon tahini

3 cloves garlic, minced

2 teaspoons oregano

Sea salt & black pepper to taste

## Directions:

Get a bowl and combine your cucumbers with your chickpeas and red onion.

Get a small bowl and whisk your lemon juice, olive oil, lemon zest, tahini, garlic, sea salt, oregano and pepper.

Toss the dressing with your salad before serving.

## Nutrition:

Calories: 231

Protein: 12 Grams

Fat: 12 Grams

Carbohydrates: 8 Grams

Sodium: 160 mg

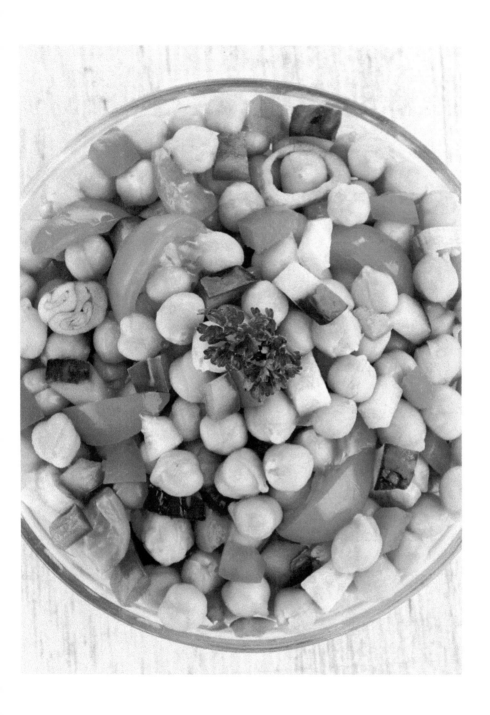

# Eggplant Rolls

**Difficulty Level: 2/5**

**Preparation time: 10 minutes**

**Cooking time: 6 minutes**

**Servings: 6**

**Ingredients:**

1 eggplant, ½ inch sliced lengthwise

Sea salt & black pepper to taste

1 tablespoon olive oil

1/3 cup cream cheese

½ cup tomatoes, chopped

1 clove garlic, minced

2 tablespoons dill, chopped

## Directions:

Slice your eggplant before brushing it down with olive oil. Season your eggplant slices with salt and pepper.

Grill the eggplants for three minutes per side.

Get out a bowl and combine cream cheese, garlic, dill and tomatoes in a different bowl.

Allow your eggplant slices to cool and then spread the mixture over each one. Roll them and pin them with a toothpick to serve.

## Nutrition:

Calories: 91

Protein: 2.1 Grams

Fat: 7 Grams

Carbohydrates: 6.3 Grams

Sodium: 140 mg

# Heavenly Quinoa

**Difficulty Level: 2/5**

**Preparation time: 15 minutes**

**Cooking time: 5 minutes**

**Servings: 5**

**Ingredients:**

1 cup almonds

1 cup quinoa

1 teaspoon cinnamon

1 pinch sea salt

1 teaspoon vanilla extract, pure

2 cups milk

2 tablespoons honey, raw

3 dates, dried, pitted & chopped fine

5 apricots, dried & chopped fine

**Directions:**

Get out a skillet to toast your almonds in for about five minutes. They should be golden and aromatic.

Place your quinoa and cinnamon in a saucepan using medium heat. Add in your vanilla, salt and milk. Stir and then bring it to a boil. Reduce your heat, and allow it to simmer for fifteen minutes.

Add in your dates, honey, apricots and half of your almonds.

Serve topped with almonds and parsley if desired.

**Nutrition:**

Calories: 344

Protein: 12.6 Grams

Fat: 13.8 Grams

Carbohydrates: 45.7 Grams

Sodium: 96 mg

# Red Bean & Green Salad

**Difficulty Level: 2/5**

**Preparation time: 10 minutes**

**Cooking time: 0 minutes**

**Servings: 6**

**Ingredients:**

1 cup red beans, cooked & drained

1 cup lettuce, shredded & chopped

2 cups spinach leaves

1 cup red onions, sliced into thin rings

½ cup walnuts, halved

3 tablespoon olive oil

3 tablespoons lemon juice, fresh

1 clove garlic, minced

1 teaspoon dijon mustard

¼ teaspoon sea salt, fine **/** ¼ teaspoon black pepper

## Directions:

Combine your lettuce, spinach, walnut, red beans and red onion together.

In a different bowl mix your olive oil, garlic, Dijon mustard and lemon juice together to form your dressing.

Drizzle the dressing over the salad and adjust salt and pepper as necessary.

Serve immediately.

## Nutrition:

Calories: 242

Protein: 10.1 Grams

Fat: 13.7 Grams

Carbohydrates: 22.7 Grams

Sodium: 121 mg

# Chickpea Patties

**Difficulty Level: 2/5**

**Preparation time: 10 minutes**

**Cooking time: 15 minutes**

**Servings: 8**

**Ingredients:**

1 Cup Flour

¾ Cup hot water

1 egg, whisked

½ teaspoon cumin

½ teaspoon sea salt, fine

1 cup spinach, fresh & chopped

3 cloves garlic, minced

1/8 teaspoon baking soda

¾ cup chickpeas, cooked

2 scallions, small & chopped

1 cup olive oil

## Directions:

Get a bowl and mix your salt, cumin and flour together. Add in your water and egg to form a batter. Whisk well. It should thicken.

Stir in your baking soda, garlic, spinach, chickpeas, and scallions, blending well.

Get a pan and place it over high heat. Add in your oil. Once your oil begins to simmer, pour in a tablespoon of your batter, frying on both sides. Repeat until all your batter is used.

Garnish with lime and greens before serving.

## Nutrition:

Calories: 352

Protein: 6.1 Grams

Fat: 27.1 Grams

Carbohydrates: 24 Grams

Sodium: 160 mg

# Red Onion Tilapia

**Difficulty Level: 2/5**

**Preparation time: 10 minutes**

**Cooking time: 5 minutes**

**Servings: 4**

**Ingredients:**

1 tablespoon olive oil

1 tablespoon orange juice, fresh

¼ teaspoon sea salt, fine

1 avocado, pitted, skinned & sliced

¼ cup red onion, chopped

4 tilapia fillets, 4 ounces each

**Directions:**

Start by getting out a pie dish that is nine inches. Glass is best. Use a fork to mix your slat, orange juice and oil together. Dip one filet at a time and then put them in your dish. They should be coated on both sides. Put them in a wheel formation so that each fillet is in the center of the dish and draped over the edge. Top each fillet with a tablespoon of onion. Fold the fillet that's hanging over your pie dish in half so that it's over the onion.

Cover it with plastic wrap but don't close it all the way. They should be able to vent the steam. Microwave for three minutes.

Tip with avocado to serve.

**Nutrition:**

Calories: 200

Protein: 22 Grams

Fat: 11 Grams

Carbohydrates: 4 Grams

Sodium: 151

# Chicken & Asparagus

**Difficulty Level: 2/5**

**Preparation time: 10 minutes**

**Cooking time: 10 minutes**

**Servings: 4**

**Ingredients:**

1 lb. Chicken breast, boneless & skinless

¼ cup flour

4 tablespoons butter

½ teaspoon sea salt, fine

½ teaspoon black pepper

1 teaspoon lemon pepper seasoning

2 slices lemon

1-2 cups asparagus, chopped

2 tablespoons honey, raw

Parsley to garnish

**Directions:**

Cover your chicken using plastic wrap and beat it until it's ¾ of an inch thick.

Get out a bowl and mix your slat, flour and pepper together. Coat your chicken in your flour mixture.

Get out a pan to melt two tablespoons of butter over medium-high heat.

Place the chicken breast in the pan to cook for three to five minutes. It should turn golden brown on each side.

While your chicken is cooking sprinkle the lemon on each side. Once it's cooked, transfer it to a plate. In the same pan add in your asparagus, cooking until it's crisp but tender. It should turn a bright green. Set it to the side.

You'll use the same pan to add your lemon slices to caramelize.

**Nutrition:**

Calories: 530

Protein: 36.8 Grams

Fat: 33.3 Grams

Carbohydrates: 28.8 Grams

Sodium: 130 mg

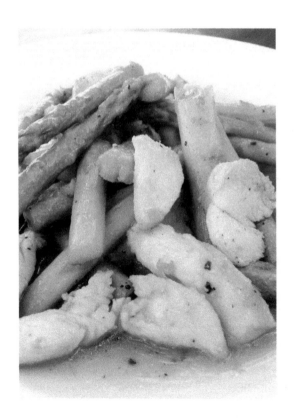

# Beef Kofta

**Difficulty Level: 2/5**

**Preparation time: 15 minutes**

**Cooking time: 15 minutes**

**Servings: 4**

**Ingredients:**

1 lb. Ground beef, 93% lean or more

½ cup onions, minced

1 tablespoon olive oil

½ teaspoon sea salt, fine

½ teaspoon coriander, ground

½ teaspoon cumin, ground

¼ teaspoon cinnamon

¼ teaspoon mint leaves, dried

¼ teaspoon allspice

## Directions:

Mix your beef, salt, cumin, coriander, cinnamon, oil, onion, mint and allspice together in a large bowl.

Get out wooden skewers and shape beef kebabs from the mixture.

Refrigerate for ten minutes before grilling them. You will need to preheat your grill and cook them for fourteen minutes. Remember to turn them constantly to avoid burning.

Serve warm.

## Nutrition:

Calories: 216

Protein: 26.1 Grams

Fat: 12.2 Grams

Carbohydrates: 1.3 Grams

Sodium: 152 mg

# Raisin Rice Pilaf

**Difficulty Level: 2/5**

**Preparation time: 5 minutes**

**Cooking time: 15 minutes**

**Servings: 4**

## Ingredients:

1 tablespoon olive oil

1 teaspoon cumin

1 cup onion, chopped

½ cup carrot, shredded

½ teaspoon cinnamon

2 cups instant brown rice

1 ¾ cup orange juice

1 cup golden raisins

¼ cup water

½ cup pistachios, shelled

Fresh Chives, Chopped for Garnish

## Directions:

Place a medium saucepan over medium-high heat before adding in your oil. Add n your onion, and stir often so it doesn't burn. Cook for about five minutes and then add in your cumin, cinnamon and carrot. Cook for about another minute.

Add in your orange juice, water and rice. Bring it all to a boil before covering your saucepan. Turn the heat down to medium-low and then allow it to simmer for six to seven minutes. Your rice should be cooked all the way through, and all the liquid should be absorbed.

Stir in your pistachios, chives and raisins. Serve warm.

## Nutrition:

Calories: 320

Protein: 6 Grams

Fat: 7 Grams

Carbohydrates: 61 Grams

Sodium: 37 mg

# Lebanese Delight

**Difficulty Level: 2/5**

**Preparation time: 5 minutes**

**Cooking time: 25 minutes**

**Servings: 5**

**Ingredients:**

1 tablespoon olive oil

1 cup vermicelli (can be substituted for thin spaghetti) broken into 1 to 1 ½ inch pieces

3 cups cabbage, shredded

3 cups vegetable broth, low sodium

½ cup water

1 cup instant brown rice

¼ teaspoon sea salt, fine

2 cloves garlic

¼ teaspoon crushed red pepper

½ cup cilantro fresh & chopped

Lemon slices to garnish

## Directions:

Get a saucepan and then place it over medium-high heat. Add in your oil and once it's hot you will need to add in your pasta. Cook for three minutes or until your pasta is toasted. You will have to stir often in order to keep it from burning.

Add in your cabbage, cooking for another four minutes. Continue to stir often.

Add in your water and rice. Season with salt, red pepper and garlic before bringing it all to a boil over high heat. Stir, and then cover. Once it's covered turn the heat down to medium-low. Allow it all to simmer for ten minutes.

Remove the pan from the burner and then allow it to sit without lifting the lid for five minutes. Take the garlic cloves out and then mash them using a fork. Place them back in, and stir them into the rice. Stir in your cilantro as well and serve warm. Garnish with lemon wedges if desired.

## Nutrition:

Calories: 259

Protein: 7 Grams

Fat: 4 Grams

Carbohydrates: 49 Grams

Sodium: 123 mg

# Flavorful Braised Kale

**Difficulty Level: 2/5**

**Preparation time: 15 minutes**

**Cooking time: 15 minutes**

**Servings: 4**

**Ingredients:**

1 lb. Kale, stems removed & chopped roughly

1 cup cherry tomatoes, halved

2 teaspoons olive oil

4 cloves garlic, sliced thin

½ cup vegetable stock

¼ teaspoon sea salt, fine

1 tablespoon lemon juice, fresh

1/8 teaspoon black pepper

## Directions:

Start by heating your olive oil in a frying pan using medium heat, and add in your garlic. Sauté for a minute or two until lightly golden.

Mix your kale and vegetable stock with your garlic, adding it to your pan.

Cover the pan and then turn the heat down to medium-low.

Allow it to cook until your kale wilts and part of your vegetable stock should be dissolved. It should take roughly five minutes.

Stir in your tomatoes and cook without a lid until your kale is tender, and then remove it from heat.

Mix in your salt, pepper and lemon juice before serving warm.


## Nutrition:

Calories: 70

Protein: 4 Grams

Fat: 0.5 Grams

Carbohydrates: 9 Grams

Sodium: 133 mg

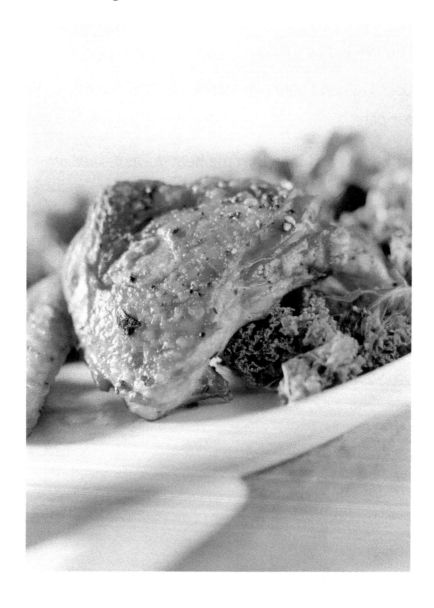

# Tomato and Wine-Steamed

# Mussels

**Difficulty Level: 2/5**

**Preparation time: 10 minutes**

**Cooking time: 15 minutes**

**Servings: 4**

**Ingredients:**

1 tablespoon olive oil

1 sweet onion, chopped

1 tablespoon minced garlic

⅛ teaspoon red pepper flakes

4 tomatoes, chopped

¼ cup low-sodium fish or chicken stock

¼ cup dry white wine

3 pounds mussels, cleaned and rinsed

Juice and zest of 1 lemon

¼ cup pitted, sliced Kalamata olives

3 tablespoons chopped fresh parsley

Sea salt

Freshly ground black pepper

## Directions:

In a large saucepan, heat the olive oil over medium-high heat. Sauté the onion, garlic, and red pepper flakes until softened, about 3 minutes. Stir in the tomatoes, stock, and wine and bring to a boil.

Add the mussels to the saucepan and cover. Steam until the mussels are opened, 6 to 7 minutes. Remove from the heat and discard any unopened shells.

Stir in the lemon juice, lemon zest, olives, and parsley. Season with salt and pepper and serve.

## Nutrition:

Calories: 162

Total fat: 7g

Saturated fat: 1g

Carbohydrates: 12g

Sugar: 5g

Fiber: 3g

Protein: 12g

# Citrus-Herb Scallops

**Difficulty Level: 2/5**

**Preparation time: 10 minutes**

**Cooking time: 4 minutes**

**Servings: 4**

**Ingredients:**

1 pound sea scallops

Sea salt

Freshly ground black pepper

2 tablespoons olive oil

Juice of 1 lime

Pinch red pepper flakes

1 tablespoon chopped fresh cilantro

## Directions:

Season the scallops lightly with salt and pepper.

In a large skillet, heat the olive oil over medium-high heat. Add the scallops to the skillet, making sure they do not touch one another.

Sear on both sides, turning once, for a total of about 3 minutes. Add the lime juice and red pepper flakes to the skillet and toss the scallops in the juice. Serve topped with cilantro.

## Nutrition:

Calories: 160

Total fat: 8g

Saturated fat: 1g

Carbohydrates: 3g

Sugar: 0g

Fiber: 0g

Protein: 19g

# Whole Baked with Lemon and Herbs

**Difficulty Level: 2/5**

**Preparation time: 10 minutes**

**Cooking time: 20 minutes**

**Servings: 4**

**Ingredients:**

1 tablespoon olive oil, divided

2 (8-ounce) whole trout, cleaned

Sea salt

Freshly ground black pepper

1 lemon, thinly sliced into about 6 pieces

1 tablespoon finely chopped fresh dill

1 tablespoon chopped fresh parsley

½ cup low-sodium fish stock or chicken stock

## Directions:

Preheat the oven to 400°F.

Lightly grease a 9-by-13-inch baking dish with 1 teaspoon of olive oil.

Rinse the trout, pat dry with paper towels, and coat with the remaining 2 teaspoons of olive oil. Season with salt and pepper.

Stuff the interior of the trout with the lemon slices, dill, and parsley and place into the prepared baking dish. Bake the fish for 10 minutes, then add the fish stock to the dish.

Continue to bake until the fish flakes easily with a fork, about 10 minutes. Serve.

## Nutrition:

Calories: 194

Total fat: 10g

Saturated fat: 2g

Carbohydrates: 1g

Sugar: 0g

Fiber: 0g

Protein: 25g

# Skillet Cod with Fresh Tomato Salsa

**Difficulty Level: 2/5**

**Preparation time: 20 minutes**

**Cooking time: 8 minutes**

**Servings: 4**

**Ingredients:**

3 tomatoes, finely chopped

1 green bell pepper, finely chopped

¼ red onion, finely chopped

¼ cup pitted, chopped green olives

2 tablespoons white wine vinegar

1 tablespoon chopped fresh basil

½ teaspoon minced garlic

4 (4-ounce) cod fillets

Sea salt

Freshly ground black pepper

1 tablespoon olive oil

**Directions:**

In a small bowl, stir together the tomatoes, bell pepper, onion, olives, vinegar, basil, and garlic until well mixed. Set aside.

Season the fish with salt and pepper.

In a large skillet, heat the olive oil over medium-high heat. Pan-fry the fish, turning once, until it is just cooked through, about 4 minutes per side.

Transfer to serving plates and top with a generous scoop of tomato salsa.

**Nutrition:**

Calories: 181

 Total fat: 7g

Saturated fat: 1g;

Carbohydrates: 9g

Sugar: 4g

Fiber: 3g

Protein: 22g

# Broiled Flounder with Nectarine and White Bean Salsa

**Difficulty Level: 2/5**

**Preparation time: 20 minutes**

**Cooking time: 8 minutes**

**Servings: 4**

## Ingredients:

2 nectarines, pitted and chopped

1 (15-ounce) can low-sodium cannellini beans, rinsed and drained

1 red bell pepper, chopped

1 scallion, both white and green parts, chopped

2 tablespoons chopped fresh cilantro

2 tablespoons freshly squeezed lime juice

4 (4-ounce) flounder fillets

1 teaspoon smoked paprika

Sea salt

Freshly ground black pepper

**Directions:**

Preheat the oven to broil.

In a medium bowl, combine the nectarines, beans, bell pepper, scallion, cilantro, and lime juice.

Season the fish with paprika, salt, and pepper.

Place the fish on a baking sheet and broil, turning once, until just cooked through, about 8 minutes total. Serve the fish topped with the salsa.

**Nutrition:**

Calories: 259

Total fat: 8g

Saturated fat: 1g

Carbohydrates: 23g

Sugar: 8g

Fiber: 7g

Protein: 26g

# Trout with Ruby Red Grapefruit Relish

**Difficulty Level: 2/5**

**Preparation time: 15 minutes**

**Cooking time: 15 minutes**

**Servings: 4**

**Ingredients:**

1 ruby red grapefruit, peeled, sectioned, and chopped

1 large navel orange, peeled, sectioned, and chopped

¼ English cucumber, chopped

2 tablespoons chopped red onion

1 tablespoon minced or grated lime zest

1 teaspoon minced fresh or canned peperoncino

1 teaspoon chopped fresh thyme

4 (4-ounce) trout fillets

Sea salt

Freshly ground black pepper

1 tablespoon olive oil

**Directions:**

Preheat the oven to 400°F.

In a medium bowl, stir together the grapefruit, orange, cucumber, onion, lime zest, peperoncino, and thyme. Cover the relish with plastic wrap and set aside in the refrigerator.

Season the trout lightly with salt and pepper and place on a baking sheet.

Brush the fish with olive oil and roast in the oven until it flakes easily with a fork, about 15 minutes. Serve topped with the chilled relish.

**Nutrition:**

Calories: 178

Total fat: 6g

Saturated fat: 1g

Carbohydrates: 10g

Sugar: 7g

Fiber: 2g

Protein: 25g

# Classic Pork Tenderloin Marsala

**Difficulty Level: 2/5**

**Preparation time: 10 minutes**

**Cooking time: 20 minutes**

**Servings: 4**

**Ingredients:**

4 (3-ounce) boneless pork loin chops, trimmed

Sea salt

Freshly ground black pepper

¼ cup whole-wheat flour

1 tablespoon olive oil

2 cups sliced button mushrooms

½ sweet onion, chopped

1 teaspoon minced garlic

½ cup Marsala wine

½ cup low-sodium chicken stock

1 tablespoon cornstarch

1 tablespoon chopped fresh parsley

**Directions:**

Lightly season the pork chops with salt and pepper.

Pour the flour onto a plate and dredge the pork chops to coat both sides, shaking off the excess.

In a large skillet, heat the olive oil over medium-high heat and pan-fry the pork chops until cooked through and browned, turning once, about 10 minutes total. Transfer the chops to a plate and set aside.

In the skillet, combine the mushrooms, onion, and garlic and sauté until the vegetables are softened, about 5 minutes.

Stir in the wine, scraping up any bits from the skillet, and bring the liquid to a simmer.

In a small bowl, stir together the stock and cornstarch until smooth. Add the stock mixture to the skillet and bring to a boil; cook, stirring, until slightly thickened, about 4 minutes. Serve the chops with the sauce, garnished with parsley.

**Nutrition:**

Calories: 200

Total fat: 6g

Saturated fat: 1g

Carbohydrates: 11g

Sugar: 1g

Fiber: 1g

Protein: 20g

# Chili-Spiced Lamb Chops

**Difficulty Level: 2/5**

**Preparation time: 2 minutes**

**Cooking time: 10 minutes**

**Servings: 4**

## Ingredients:

4 (4-ounce) loin lamb chops with bones, trimmed

Sea salt

Freshly ground black pepper

1 tablespoon olive oil

2 tablespoons Sriracha sauce

1 tablespoon chopped fresh cilantro

**Directions:**

Preheat the oven to 450°F.

Lightly season the lamb chops with salt and pepper.

In a large ovenproof skillet, heat the olive oil over medium-high heat. Brown the chops on both sides, about 2 minutes per side, and spread the chops with sriracha.

Place the skillet in the oven and roast until the desired doneness, 4 to 5 minutes for medium. Serve topped with cilantro.

**Nutrition:**

Calories: 223

Total fat: 14g

Saturated fat: 4g

Carbohydrates: 1g

Sugar: 1g

Fiber: 0g

Protein: 23g

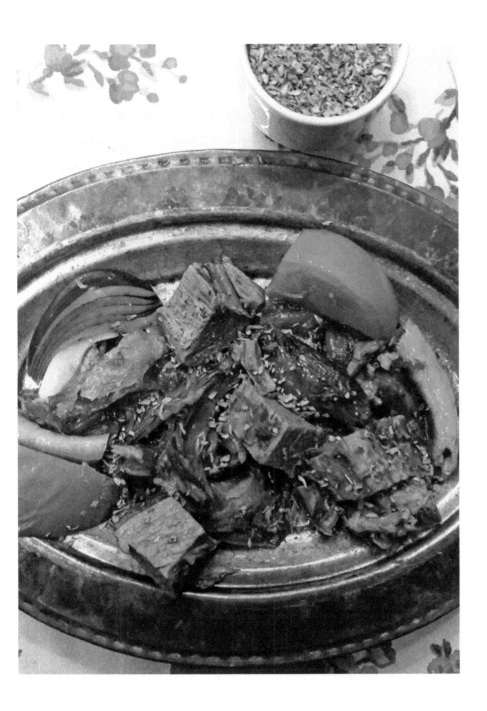

# Greek Herbed Beef Meatballs

**Difficulty Level: 3/5**

**Preparation time: 10 minutes**

**Cooking time: 20 minutes**

**Servings: 4**

**Ingredients:**

1 pound extra-lean ground beef

½ cup panko breadcrumbs

¼ cup grated Parmesan cheese

¼ cup low-fat milk

2 large eggs

1 tablespoon chopped fresh parsley

1 teaspoon chopped fresh oregano

1 teaspoon minced garlic

¼ teaspoon freshly ground black pepper

Sea salt

## Directions:

Preheat the oven to 400°F.

In a large bowl, combine the ground beef, breadcrumbs, Parmesan cheese, milk, eggs, parsley, oregano, garlic, and pepper. Season lightly with salt.

Roll the beef mixture into 1-inch meatballs and arrange on a baking sheet.

Bake the meatballs until they are cooked through and browned, turning them several times, about 20 minutes. Serve with a sauce such as Marinara Sauce or stuffed into a pita.

## Nutrition:

Calories: 243

Total fat: 8g

Saturated fat: 3g

Carbohydrates: 13g

Sugar: 1g

Fiber: 2g

Protein: 24g

# Sautéed Dark Leafy Greens

**Difficulty Level: 2/5**

**Preparation time: 10 minutes**

**Cooking time: 10 minutes**

**Servings: 4**

**Ingredients:**

2 tablespoons olive oil

8 cups stemmed and coarsely chopped spinach, kale, collard greens, or Swiss chard

Juice of ½ lemon

Sea salt

Freshly ground black pepper

**Directions:**

In a large skillet, heat the olive oil over medium-high heat. Add the greens and toss with tongs until wilted and tender, 8 to 10 minutes.

Remove the skillet from the heat and squeeze in the lemon juice, tossing to coat evenly. Season with salt and pepper and serve.

**Nutrition:**

Calories: 129

Total fat: 7g

Saturated fat: 1g

Carbohydrates: 14g

Sugar: 0g

Fiber: 2g

Protein: 4g

# Broiled Tomatoes with Feta

**Difficulty Level: 2/5**

**Preparation time: 10 minutes**

**Cooking time: 8 minutes**

**Servings: 4**

**Ingredients:**

4 large tomatoes, cut in half horizontally

1 tablespoon olive oil

1 teaspoon minced garlic

½ cup crumbled feta cheese

1 tablespoon chopped fresh basil

Sea salt

Freshly ground black pepper

## Directions:

Preheat the oven to broil.

Place the tomato halves, cut-side up, in a 9-by-13-inch baking dish and drizzle them with the olive oil. Rub the garlic into the tomatoes.

Broil the tomatoes for about 5 minutes, until softened. Sprinkle with the feta cheese and broil for 3 minutes longer.

Sprinkle with basil and season with salt and pepper. Serve.

## Nutrition:

Calories: 113

Total fat: 8g

Saturated fat: 3g

Carbohydrates: 8g

Sugar: 6g

Fiber: 2g

Protein: 4g

# Mediterranean Lamb Chops

**Difficulty Level: 2/5**

**Preparation time: 10 minutes**

**Cooking time: 10 minute**

**Servings: 4**

## Ingredients

4 lamb shoulder chops, 8 ounce each

2 tablespoons Dijon mustard

2 tablespoons Balsamic vinegar

1 tablespoon garlic, chopped

½ cup olive oil

2 tablespoons shredded fresh basil

## Directions:

Pat your lamb chop dry using kitchen towel and arrange them on a shallow glass baking dish.

Take a bowl and whisk in Dijon mustard, balsamic vinegar, garlic, pepper and mix well.

Whisk in the oil very slowly into the marinade until the mixture is smooth.

Stir in basil.

Pour the marinade over the lamb chops and stir to coat both sides well.

Cover the chops and allow them to marinate for 1-4 hours (chilled).

Take the chops out and leave them for 30 minutes to allow the temperature to reach normal level.

Pre-heat your grill to medium heat and add oil to the grate.

Grill the lamb chops for 5-10 minutes per side until both sides are browned.

Once the center of the chop reads 145 degree Fahrenheit, the chops are ready, serve and enjoy!

**Nutrition** (Per Serving)

Calories: 521

Fat: 45g

Carbohydrates: 3.5g

Protein: 22g

# Broiled Mushrooms Burgers and Goat Cheese

**Difficulty Level: 2/5**

**Preparation time: 15 minutes**

**Cooking time: 5 minutes**

**Servings: 4**

**Ingredients:**

4 large Portobello mushroom caps

1 red onion, cut into ¼ inch thick slices

2 tablespoons extra virgin olive oil

2 tablespoons balsamic vinegar

Pinch of salt

¼ cup goat cheese

¼ cup sun-dried tomatoes, chopped

4 ciabatta buns

1 cup kale, shredded

**Directions:**

Pre-heat your oven to broil.

Take a large bowl and add mushrooms caps, onion slices, olive oil, balsamic vinegar and salt.

Mix well.

Place mushroom caps (bottom side up) and onion slices on your baking sheet.

Take a small bowl and stir in goat cheese and sun dried tomatoes.

Toast the buns under the broiler for 30 seconds until golden.

Spread the goat cheese mix on top of each bun.

Place mushroom cap and onion slice on each bun bottom and cover with shredded kale.

Put everything together and serve.

Enjoy!

**Nutrition** (Per Serving)

Calories: 327

Fat: 11g

Carbohydrates: 49g

Protein: 11g

# Garlic Rice

**Difficulty Level: 2/5**

**Preparation time: 5 minutes**

**Cooking time: 3 minutes**

**Servings: 4**

**Ingredients**

2 tablespoons vegetable oil

1 1/2 tablespoons chopped garlic

2 tablespoons ground pork

4 cups cooked white rice

1 1/2 teaspoons of garlic salt

ground black pepper to taste

**Directions:**

Heat the oil in a large frying pan over medium heat. When the oil is hot, add the garlic and ground pork. Boil and stir until garlic is golden brown.

Stir in cooked white rice and season with garlic salt and pepper. Bake and stir until the mixture is hot and well mixed for about 3 minutes.

**Nutrition:** (Per Serving)

Calories 293;

Fat 9 g;

Carbohydrates 45.9 g;

Protein 5.9 g

Cholesterol 6 mg;

Sodium 686 mg

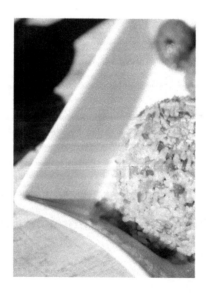

# Peppered Shrimp

**Difficulty Level: 2/5**

**Preparation time: 5 minutes**

**Cooking time: 20 minutes**

**Servings: 6**

## Ingredients

12 kg penne

1/4 cup butter

2 tablespoons extra virgin olive oil

1 onion, diced

2 cloves of chopped garlic

1 red pepper, diced

1/2 kg Portobello mushrooms, cubed

1 pound shrimp, peeled and thawed

1 jar of Alfredo sauce

1/2 cup of grated Romano cheese

1/2 cup of cream

1/4 cup chopped parsley

1 teaspoon cayenne pepper

salt and pepper to taste

## Directions:

Bring a large pot of lightly salted water to a boil. Put the pasta and cook for 8 to 10 minutes or until al dente; drain.

Meanwhile, melt the butter and olive oil in a pan over medium heat. Stir in the onion and cook until soft and translucent, about 2 minutes. Stir in garlic, red pepper and mushrooms; cook over medium heat until soft, about 2 minutes longer.

Stir in the shrimp and fry until firm and pink, then add Alfredo sauce, Romano cheese and cream; bring to a boil, constantly stirring until thick, about 5 minutes. Season with cayenne pepper, salt, and pepper to taste. Add the drained pasta to the sauce and sprinkle with chopped parsley.

**Nutrition:** (Per Serving)

707 calories;

45 g fat;

50.6 g carbohydrates;

28.4 g of protein;

201 mg of cholesterol;

1034 mg of sodium.

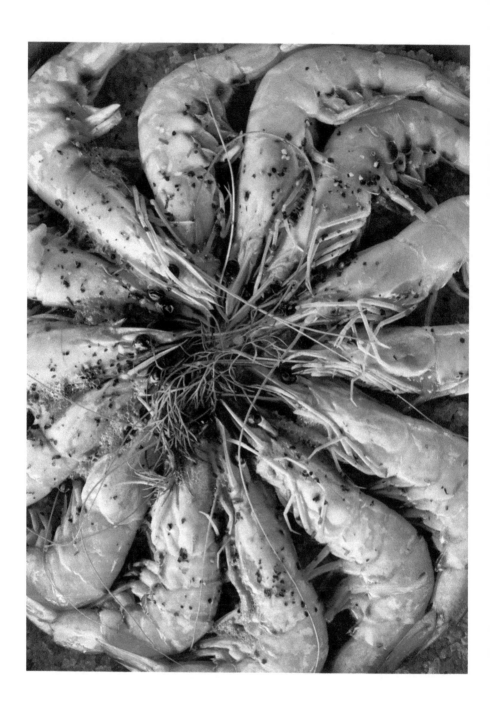